CHESTNUTS for the MRCP

differential diagnoses in medicine

D0715979

Published by ReMEDICA Publishing Limited
32–38 Osnaburgh Street, London, NW1 3ND, UK

Tel: +44 207 388 7677
Fax: +44 207 388 7457
Email: books@remedica.com
www.remedica.com

Publisher: Andrew Ward
In-house editors: Charissa Deane and Tamsin White
Design: ReGRAPHICA, London, UK

ISBN 1 901346 39 0
British Library Cataloguing-in Publication Data
A catalogue record for this book is available from the British Library

CHESTNUTS for the MRCP

differential diagnoses in medicine

Levy MJ
Porter WM

ReMEDICAPUBLISHING

Dedicated to Ratty

Contents

Foreword

This book is not designed to be easy reading. It is simply a catalogue of lists that have been amalgamated by previous MRCP candidates who have sat the Part 1 and Part 2 examinations. The lists, or 'Chestnuts', contain a collection of important differential diagnoses that are relevant to clinical practice and both parts of the MRCP exam. The lists will enable you to create useful differential diagnoses on the spot. It is hoped that these lists will provide you with a concise and portable text that will be continually relevant to the examination, as well as clinical medicine.

The book has two parts. Part A consists of important lists relevant to each speciality. Ideally, these lists should be committed to memory. There is space in the book for you to add further information or aide-mémoires. Part B contains lists of the most frequently encountered diagnoses in the Membership. Underneath each diagnosis is an amalgamation of the relevant data from Part A.

The book has been designed so that you can carry it around at all times. Having these lists at close hand will hopefully provide you with a reassuring reference to consult in the final run up to both the written and clinical parts of the exam. The hunger for knowledge should be enough to motivate you to go through the pain of learning these lists. Unfortunately, lists can only be learned by active transport rather than osmosis! Experienced MRCP examiners often say that the outstanding candidates are the ones who can vocalise differential diagnoses effortlessly.

The Chestnuts are in no way exhaustive and should be extended as you feel necessary. The differing lists in Parts A and B will allow you to make lateral connections across different specialities, which is a very useful skill to possess both in examinations and in clinical practice.

Whilst being a valuable revision tool for MRCP examinations, these lists will help medical students pass and excel in their finals. This book should also be in the hands of all physicians who wish to continue to impress their colleagues in clinics, meetings and on ward rounds throughout their career!

Dr Miles Levy MBBS MRCP
Specialist Registrar General Medicine and Endocrinology, Clinical Research Fellow Neuroendocrinology,
National Hospital for Neurology and Neurosurgery, Queen Square, London, UK

Dr William Porter MBBS MRCP
Consultant Dermatologist,
Gloucestershire Royal Hospital, UK

How to Use This Book

Part A

Ideally you should learn every list in this section of the book—it is rather a tall order but it will put you at a considerable advantage over your colleagues if you do.

If you are an MRCP candidate then you should memorise as much of each list as possible. If you are a finals candidate, generally the first four entries will be the most important. If you are on the wards or in clinic, then keep it close at hand so that you can refer to it at any time.

You should cover up each stem until you can recite the complete list. It will take approximately 3 months to learn it all, so start early. Once the lists have been memorised they will be in the back of your mind throughout your career, so it is worth the effort if you are planning on being a physician who can hold his/her own in general medicine.

The book is yours and therefore you should feel free to write your own aide-mémoires. If you feel that an important part of a list has not been included then add it yourself beside the relevant one.

If you think the list is too long and only a certain number of entries need to be memorised, then add your own edited list beside it. The act of physically writing your own list makes memorising it easier.

If you disagree with any of the lists, it is important that you change them to your own preference.

Part B

It is not essential to memorise this section of the book. The best way of using this section is to systematically go through each member of the list so that you familiarise yourself with the combination of signs and investigation findings that may unify a single diagnosis. Often in medical exams (and clinical practice) a unifying diagnosis is not immediately obvious but the penny may drop if you consult these lists when given a case history with lots of data that do not seem to be related.

The other way of using this section is to test yourself as you are going through each list. Each member of the list in section B is the head of a stem in section A that you may have previously memorised. If you use both parts in combination you will start to recognise patterns and make sensible diagnoses.

These lists are not a replacement for understanding the pathophysiology and management of disease. However, clinical acumen develops with experience and pattern recognition which, unless you've been around for years, can only be expedited by books such as this!

Acidosis: normal anion gap

Renal tubular acidosis
Ureterosigmoidostomy
Biliary fistula
Acetazolamide
Fulminant diarrhoea

Acidosis: raised anion gap

With hypoxia
Sepsis
Congestive cardiac failure
Leukaemia
Anaemia
Haemorrhage
Without hypoxia
Methanol
Ethylene glycol
Metformin
Salicylates
Diabetic ketoacidosis
Renal failure
Liver failure
G6PD deficiency

Alpha-fetoprotein: raised

Hepatoma
Germ cell tumour
Carcinoma
Emphysema
Cirrhosis
Fetus with Down syndrome

Amyloidosis

AA
Chronic inflammatory disease
Chronic infection
Malignancy
AL
Myeloma
Lymphoma
Macroglobulinaemia
Monoclonal gammopathy

Clinitest positive

Glucose
Lactose
Galactose
Salicylates
Homogentisic acid (alkaptonuria)

Creatine kinase: raised

Myocardial infarction
Rhabdomyolysis
Rigorous exercise
Hyperpyrexia
Myositis
Burns
Hypothyroidism
Azathioprine
Muscular dystrophy
Alcohol

Creatinine/urea: raised

Rhabdomyolysis
Liver failure
Trimethoprim
Cimetidine
Dialysis
Pregnancy
Racial variation

Fanconi's syndrome

Congenital
Cystinosis
Galactosaemia
Wilson's disease
Acquired
Drugs
Dysproteinaemias
Heavy metals

Ferritin: raised

Acute phase response
Thalassaemia
Iron therapy
Haemochromatosis
Sideroblastic anaemia

Homocysteinuria

Autosomal recessive
Downward lens displacement
Osteoporosis
Thrombosis
Low IQ

Hyperaldosteronism

Conn's adenoma
Bilateral adrenal hyperplasia
Glucocorticoid-remediable hyperaldosteronism
Adrenal carcinoma

Hypercalcaemia

Malignancy
Hyperparathyroidism
Sarcoidosis
Vitamin D excess
Familial hypocalciuric hypercalcaemia
Hypoadrenalism
Myeloma
Diuretics
Thyrotoxicosis
Milk-alkali syndrome (excess antacids)

Metabolism

Hyperkalaemia

Renal failure
Hypoadrenalism
Hypoaldosteronism
Haemolysed blood sample
Familial pseudohyperkalaemia
Drugs
Trauma
Surgery
Burns
Tumour lysis syndrome

Hyperlipidaemia: secondary

Alcohol
Diabetes
Steroids
Hypothyroidism
Obstructive jaundice
Nephrotic syndrome
Thiazides
Contraceptive pill (combined)

Hypermagnesaemia

Renal failure
Burns
Rhabdomyolysis
Diabetic ketoacidosis

Hypernatraemia

Hypotonic fluid loss
Hyperosmolar non-ketotic coma
Iatrogenic
Reduced water intake

Hyperphosphataemia

Renal failure
Rhabdomyolysis
Hypoparathyroidism
Pseudohypoparathyroidism

Hypoalbuminaemia

Malnutrition
Malabsorption
Protein losing enteropathy
Renal loss
Liver disease
Malignancy
Catabolic state

Hypocalcaemia

Vitamin D deficiency
Chronic renal failure
Malabsorption
Magnesium deficiency
Hypoparathyroidism
Rhabdomyolysis
Pancreatitis
Phosphate binders
Chemotherapy

Hypoglycaemia

Fasting
Insulinoma
Hypopituitarism
Addison's disease
Cirrhosis
Sarcoma
Insulin
Sulphonylureas
Sepsis
Insulin stimulating antibodies
Non-fasting
Early diabetes mellitus
Gastric surgery

Metabolism

Hypokalaemic alkalosis

Diuretics
Cushing's syndrome
Conn's syndrome
Bartter's syndrome
Carbenoxolone
Purgatives
Villous adenoma of rectum
Excess antacid ingestion
Liddle's syndrome
Ureterosigmoidostomy
Purgative abuse
β_2 agonists

Hypomagnesaemia

Malabsorption
Diuretics
Cisplatinum
Gentamicin
Hyperthyroidism
Post-acute tubular necrosis
Pancreatitis
Hypercalcaemia

Hyponatraemia
Na/H_2O retention
Congestive cardiac failure
Nephrotic syndrome
Cirrhosis
Renal artery stenosis
Hypothyroidism
Na loss
Diuretics
Hypoadrenalism
Diarrhoea/vomiting
Salt-losing nephritis
Pure H_2O retention
Iatrogenic
Psychogenic polydipsia
Syndrome of inappropriate ADH

Hypophosphataemia

Hyperparathyroidism
X-linked hypophosphataemic rickets
Idiopathic
Dialysis
Vitamin D deficiency
Chelating drugs in renal failure
Burns
Fanconi's syndrome
Liver failure

Lag-storage curve with glucose tolerance test

Normal variant
Gastrectomy
Diabetes
Liver disease
Thyrotoxicosis

Syndrome of inappropriate ADH

Cancer
Lung
Leukaemia/lymphoma
Pancreas
CNS
Cerebral abscess
Neurosarcoidosis
Haemorrhage
Meningioma
Intracranial pressure: raised
Guillain Barré syndrome
Respiratory
Empyema
Abscess
Bronchial carcinoma
Lung fibrosis
Tuberculosis
Ventilation
Metabolic
Acute intermittent porphyria

Urate: raised
Increased production
Gout
Psoriasis
Myeloproliferative disease
Lymphoproliferative disease
Polycythaemia
Lesch-Nyhan syndrome
Reduced excretion
Renal impairment
Hyperparathyroidism
Diuretics
Gout
Hypothyroidism
Pre-eclampsia
Familial

Urea/creatinine: raised

Sepsis
Haemorrhage
Pre-renal renal failure
Hypoadrenalism
Acute or chronic renal failure
Steroids
Old tetracyclines

Endocrinology

Active vs. inactive acromegaly

Headache
Sweating
Soft tissue swelling/nerve compression
Hypertension
Diabetes mellitus

Androgenisation

Polycystic ovarian syndrome
Congenital adrenal hyperplasia
Cushing's syndrome
Adrenal tumours

Childhood obesity

Lawrence-Moon-Biedle syndrome
Prader-Willi syndrome
Leptin deficiency
Alström's syndrome

Cushing's syndrome

Pituitary-driven (Cushing's disease)
Adrenal tumour
Ectopic adrenocorticotropic hormone
Exogenous steroids

Diabetes insipidus

Cranial
Tumour
Surgery
Trauma
Ischaemia
Sarcoidosis
Histiocytosis X
Lymphocytic hypophysitis
DIDMOAD
Nephrogenic
Hypercalcaemia
Hypokalaemia
Lithium
X-linked
Renal failure

Dynamic tests

Hormone excess
Acromegaly: glucose tolerance test
Cushing's: dexamethasone suppression test
Testosterone: dexamethasone suppression test
Hormone deficiency
Growth hormone: insulin tolerance test/glucagon test
ACTH: insulin tolerance test
LH/FSH: GnRH stimulation test
TSH: TRH stimulation test
Cortisol: synacthen test

Galactorrhoea

Pregnancy
Prolactinoma
Pituitary mass lesion ('stalk effect')
Anti-dopaminergic drugs
Oestrogen
Chronic renal failure
Hypothyroidism
Ectopic prolactin (kidney, lung tumours)

Gynaecomastia

Drugs
Digoxin
Spironolactone
Chlorpromazine
Methyldopa
Cimetidine
Miscellaneous
Bronchial carcinoma
Liver disease
Klinefelter's syndrome
Dialysis
Acromegaly
Lymphoma
Oestrogen-producing tumours

Hypercortisolaemia

Pregnancy
Cushing's syndrome
Stress
Alcohol
Obesity
Depression

Hyperprolactinaemia

Prolactinoma
Non-functioning adenoma ('stalk effect')
Cirrhosis
Hypothyroidism
Chronic renal failure
Anti-dopaminergic drugs

Hypoadrenalism

Primary
Autoimmune
Tuberculosis
Adrenal haemorrhage
Sarcoidosis
Amyloid
HIV
Haemochromatosis
Adrenalectomy
Secondary
Pituitary disease
Isolated ACTH deficiency
Steroid withdrawal

Hypopituitarism

Tumour
Surgery
Radiotherapy
Congenital
Pituitary apoplexy
Infiltrative disease

Hypothyroidism

Primary
Autoimmune
Post-partum
Radioactive iodine
Anti-thyroid drugs
Amiodarone
Lithium
Iodine deficiency
Congenital
Secondary
Pituitary disease
TSH/T4 resistance

Multiple endocrine neoplasia type 1

Pituitary
Pancreatic
Parathyroid
PPP

Multiple endocrine neoplasia type 2

Phaeochromocytoma
Medullary Ca thyroid
Parathyroid
PHAMPAR

Noonan's syndrome

Same appearance as Turner's
Pulmonary stenosis
Normal fertility

Obesity and hypogonadism

Edward's syndrome
Prader-Willi syndrome
Lawrence-Moon-Biedle syndrome

Endocrinology

Short stature

Proportional
Growth hormone deficiency
Systemic disease
Constitutional delay
Familial
Disproportional
Turner's syndrome
Achondroplasia
Osteogenesis imperfecta
Congenital hypothyroidism

Testosterone low

Primary
Klinefelter's syndrome
Testicular tumour
Testicular agenesis
Torsion
Maldescent
Steroid enzyme deficiencies
Drugs
Secondary
Pituitary disease
Isolated GnRH deficiency
Kallmann's syndrome
Anorexia nervosa

Thyrotoxicosis

Grave's disease
Multinodular goitre
Single toxic nodule
Drugs e.g. amiodarone
Thyroxine over-use
Ovarian tumours
TSHoma

Turner's syndrome: associations

Coarctation of aorta
Ventriculoseptal defect
Osteoporosis
Lymphoedema

Nephrology

Calcification of kidney

Diffuse
Hyperparathyroidism
Sarcoidosis
Medullary sponge kidney
Renal tubular acidosis
Miliary tuberculosis
Local
Haematoma
Histoplasmosis
Focal tuberculosis
Renal carcinoma
Hydatid cyst

Chronic renal failure vs. acute renal failure

Neuropathy
Pruritis
Osteodystrophy
Anaemia
Small kidneys

Congenital renal disease

Adult polycystic kidney disease
Medullary sponge kidney
Medullary cystic kidney
Nephrogenic diabetes insipidus (X-linked)
Alport's syndrome
Renal tubular disorders
Fabry's disease
Familial IgA nephropathy

Enlarged kidney (unilateral)

Hydronephrosis
Adult polycystic kidney disease
Renal carcinoma
Congenital anomaly

IgA nephropathy: associations

Post-upper respiratory tract infection
Gastroenteritis
Urinary tract infection
Henoch-Schönlein purpura
Coeliac disease

Interstitial nephritis: drugs

Non-steroidal anti-inflammatory drugs
Rifampicin
Warfarin
Allopurinol
Omeprazole

Nephrotic syndrome

Glomerulonephritis
Vasculitis
Sickle cell anaemia
Malaria
Gold
Penicillamine
Vesico-ureteric reflux
Amyloidosis
Constrictive pericarditis
Pre-eclampsia

Nephrotic syndrome: complications

Thrombosis
Sepsis
Hyperlipidaemia
Renal failure
Protein malnutrition

Osteomalacia

Malabsorption
Diet
Renal failure
Anticonvulsants
Renal tubular acidosis
Vitamin D resistant rickets

Osteoporosis

Endocrine
Cushing's syndrome
Thyrotoxicosis
Hypogonadism
Acromegaly
Prolactinoma
Congenital
Turner's syndrome
Osteogenesis imperfecta
Homocystinuria
Drugs
Alcohol
Heparin
Steroids
Miscellaneous
Rheumatoid arthritis
Scurvy
Paget's disease
Idiopathic

Polycystic kidneys: associations

Polycythaemia
Berry aneurysms
Mitral valve prolapse
Hepatic cysts

Pyuria

Non-steroidal anti-inflammatory drugs
Urinary tract infection
Medullary sponge kidney
Interstitial nephritis
Hypokalaemia
Nephrocalcinosis

Renal failure and low complement

Systemic lupus erythematosus
Bacterial endocarditis
Shunt nephritis
Mixed essential cryoglobulinaemia
Mesangiocapillary glomerulonephritis
Cholesterol embolus

Renal failure and myeloma

Hypercalcaemia
Bence Jones proteins
Hyperviscosity
Chemotherapy
Hyperuricaemia

Renal failure with normal/large size kidneys

Polycystic kidneys
Amyloidosis
Sarcoidosis
Diabetes
Lymphoma
Myeloma

Renal failure and sarcoidosis

Hypercalcaemia
Hypercalciuria
Renal granulomas
Glomerulonephritis

Renal papillary necrosis

Non-steroidal anti-inflammatory drugs
Sickle cell anaemia
Diabetes
Tuberculosis
Dysproteinaemias
Pyelonephritis
Gout

Renal scarring

Reflux nephropathy
Obstructive uropathy
Renal papillary necrosis

Salt-losing nephritis

Pyelonephritis
Renal papillary necrosis
Relief of obstructive uropathy
Recovery of acute tubular necrosis
Adult polycystic kidney disease

Gastroenterology

Abdominal pain and renal impairment

Hypercalcaemia
Vasculitis
Abdominal malignancy
Retroperitoneal pathology
Sepsis

Abdominal pain (non-surgical)

Diabetic ketoacidosis
Addison's disease
Hepatitis
Sickle crisis
Acute intermittent porphyria
Lead poisoning
Familial Mediterranean fever
Paroxysmal nocturnal haemoglobinuria

Aphthous ulceration

Crohn's disease
Reiter's disease
Coeliac disease
Trauma
Folate deficiency
Behcet's syndrome

Ascites

Cirrhosis
Congestive cardiac failure
Nephrotic syndrome
Malignancy
Budd-Chiari syndrome
Portal vein thrombosis
Tuberculous peritonitis
Constrictive pericarditis
Ovarian hyperstimulation syndrome
Peritoneal mesothelioma

Bacterial overgrowth

Hypochlorhydria
Bowel surgery
Fistula
Diverticula
Systemic sclerosis
Amyloid
Autonomic neuropathy

Budd-Chiari syndrome

Thrombophilia
Malignancy
Pregnancy
Drugs
Hepatic infection
Trauma

Chronic liver disease

Viral hepatitis
Alcohol
Autoimmune
Primary biliary cirrhosis
Wilson's disease
Alpha-1 antitrypsin deficiency
Haemochromatosis
Drugs

Coeliac disease: associations

Gastrointestinal malignancies
T-cell lymphoma
Myopathy
Neuropathy
Hyposplenism
Dermatitis herpetiformis

Congenital hyperbilirubinaemia

Conjugated
Dubin-Johnson syndrome
Rotor's syndrome
Unconjugated
Gilbert's disease
Crigler-Najjar syndrome

Congenital liver disease

Haemochromatosis
Wilson's disease
Primary biliary cirrhosis
Alpha-1 antitrypsin deficiency
Reye's syndrome

Crohn's disease: associations

Erythema nodosum
Episcleritis
Uveitis
Chronic active hepatitis
Amyloidosis
Gall stones
Arthropathy

Gastrectomy: complications

Dumping syndrome
Iron deficiency
B12/folate deficiency
Achlorhydria
Malabsorption
Osteoporosis
Osteomalacia
Gall stones
Renal stones (oxalate)

Gingival hypertrophy

Drugs
Phenytoin
Cyclosporin
Oral contraceptive pill
Nifedipine
Miscellaneous
Pregnancy
Acute myelomonocytic leukaemia
Familial
Tuberous sclerosis

Hepatic granulomas

Tuberculosis
Sarcoidosis
Primary biliary cirrhosis
Biliary obstruction
Inflammatory bowel disease
HIV
Cytomegalovirus
Epstein Barr virus
Fungal infection

Isolated hepatomegaly

Liver metastases
Congestive cardiac failure
Hepatitis
Primary biliary cirrhosis
Sarcoidosis
Haemochromatosis
Hepatoma

Macroglossia

Down syndrome
Amyloidosis
Acromegaly
Congenital hypothyroidism

Malabsorption

Infection
Inflammatory bowel disease
Bowel surgery
Irradiation
Small bowel neoplasia
Amyloid
Blind loop
Coeliac disease
Whipple's disease
Tropical sprue
Pancreatic pathology
Biliary pathology
Drugs
Endocrinopathies

Pancreatitis

Gallstones
Ethanol
Trauma
Surgery to biliary tree
Mumps
Azathioprine
Steroids
Hypothermia
Endoscopic retrograde cholangio-pancreatography
Drugs
GETSMASHED

Parotid swelling: bilateral

Mumps
Tuberculosis
Syphilis
Sarcoidosis
Alcohol
Lymphoma
Diabetes
Amyloidosis
HIV

Portal hypertension

Venous obstruction
Budd-Chiari syndrome
Right heart failure
Pericarditis
Hepatic
Cirrhosis
Chronic active hepatitis
Alcoholic hepatitis
High output
Massive splenomegaly
Arterio-venous fistula

Primary sclerosing cholangitis: associations

Ulcerative colitis
Chronic pancreatitis
Retroperitoneal fibrosis
HIV
Sjögren's syndrome
Histiocytosis X

Protein losing enteropathy

Neoplastic
Carcinoma of colon
Lymphoma
Inflammatory/infective
Crohn's/ulcerative colitis
Coeliac disease
Tropical sprue
Whipple's disease
HIV
Villous adenoma rectum
Lymphangiectasia
Primary
Cardiac/pericardial disease
Abdominal malignancy
Tuberculous peritonitis

Retroperitoneal fibrosis

Lymphoma
Abdominal aortic aneurysm
Radiotherapy
Carcinoid syndrome
Drugs (see Therapeutics)

Splenic calcification

Infarction
Haemangioma
Tuberculosis
Brucella
Histoplasmosis

Splenomegaly: massive

Chronic granulocytic leukaemia
Myelofibrosis
Malaria
Leishmaniasis
Gaucher's disease

Ulcerative colitis: associations

Erythema nodosum
Primary sclerosing cholangitis
Pyoderma gangrenosum
Uveitis
Episcleritis
Venous thrombosis
Ankylosing spondylitis
Cholangiocarcinoma

Haematology

Acanthocytosis

Abetalipoproteinaemia
Liver failure
Anorexia
Hypothyroidism
Amyotrophic chorea-acanthocytosis

Anisocytosis: variation in size

Iron deficiency
Megaloblastic anaemia
Thalassaemia

Atypical lymphocytosis

Viral
Epstein Barr virus
Cytomegalovirus
Toxoplasmosis
Varicella Zoster virus
Hepatitis A
HIV
Parvovirus
Rubella
Non-viral
Tuberculosis
Drugs
Systemic lupus erythematosus
Sarcoidosis

B12 deficiency

Dietary deficiency
Pernicious anaemia
Gastric disease
Malabsorption
Drugs

Basophilic stippling

Lead poisoning
Thalassaemia
Haemoglobinopathies
Sideroblastic anaemia
Pyrimidine-5'-nucleotidase deficiency

Bone marrow failure

Aplastic anaemia
Myelodysplastic syndrome
Myelofibrosis
Marrow infiltration
Leukaemia
Lymphoma
Lipid storage disease
Amyloid
Sepsis

Burr cells

Pyruvate kinase deficiency
Post-transfusion
Gastric carcinoma
Renal failure

Dilutional anaemia

2nd/3rd trimester pregnancy
Cirrhosis
Congestive cardiac failure
Splenomegaly

Dimorphic blood film

Sideroblastic anaemia
Post-gastrectomy
Mixed B12 or folate and iron deficiency
Blood transfusion
Liver disease
Partially treated iron deficiency

Disseminated intravascular coagulation

Carcinomatosis
Acute myeloid leukaemia
Sepsis
Obstetric emergencies
Trauma
Malaria
Transfusion reaction
Burns
Fat embolism
Snake venom

Eosinophilia

Parasitic infections
Allergies
Pulmonary eosinophilia
Malignancy
Lymphoma
Leukaemia
Hypoadrenalism
Löffler's syndrome
Drugs

Folate deficiency

Dietary deficiency
Malabsorption
Pregnancy
Malignancy
Drugs
Psoriasis

Haemolytic anaemia: Coombe's negative

Paroxysmal nocturnal haemoglobinuria
Artificial heart valve
Transfusion
Infection
Burns
G6PD deficiency

Haemolytic anaemia:
Coombe's positive (autoimmune)

Lymphoma
Chronic lymphocytic leukaemia
Carcinomatosis
Systemic lupus erythematosus
Epstein Barr virus
Drugs
Paroxysmal cold haemoglobinuria

Heinz bodies: blue bodies of denatured Hb

Haemolytic anaemia
G6PD deficiency
Unstable haemoglobins (e.g. Hb Koln)
Post-splenectomy

Howell-Jolly bodies

Post-splenectomy
Hyposplenism
Iron deficiency
Megaloblastic anaemia
Leukaemia

Hyposplenism

Sickle cell disease
Coeliac disease
Dermatitis herpetiformis
Ulcerative colitis
Essential thrombocythaemia
Fanconi's anaemia
Amyloidosis
Tropical sprue

Iron overload

Repeated blood transfusions
Haemochromatosis
Thalassaemia
Sideroblastic anaemia
Iron therapy

Leukaemoid reaction

Severe infection
Tuberculosis
Malignant infiltration of bone marrow
Haemolysis
Haemorrhage

Leukoerythroblastic anaemia

Tuberculous infiltration
Megaloblastic anaemia
Sarcoidosis
Myeloma
Lymphoma
Osteopetrosis

Macrocytosis

B12 deficiency
Folate deficiency
Haemolysis
Haemorrhage
Alcohol
Hypothyroidism
Drugs (see Therapeutics)
Pregnancy
Myelodysplasia
Lead poisoning

Methaemoglobinaemia

Drugs (oxidising agents)
Primaquine
Quinolones
Dapsone
Sulphasalazine
Nitrates/nitrites
Congenital

Micro-angiopathic haemolytic anaemia

Burns
Sepsis
Haemolytic uraemic syndrome
Thrombotic thrombocytopenic purpura
Carcinomatosis
Pre-eclampsia
Malignant hypertension

Microcytosis

Thalassaemia
Iron deficiency
Aluminium toxicity
Hereditary sideroblastic anaemia

Normochromic normocytic anaemia

Chronic disease
Renal failure
Hypothyroidism
Aplastic anaemia
Primary bone marrow disease

Pancytopenia

Aplastic anaemia
Hypersplenism
Paroxysmal nocturnal haemoglobinuria
Marrow infiltration
Sepsis
Systemic lupus erythematosus
Megaloblastic anaemia

Pancytopenia and raised mean corpuscular volume

B12 deficiency
Folate deficiency
Systemic lupus erythematosus
Myelodysplasia
Drugs
Paroxysmal nocturnal haemoglobinuria

Pappenheimer bodies: granules of siderocytes

Sideroblastic anaemia
Haemolytic anaemia
Post-splenectomy

Paraproteinaemias

Multiple myeloma
Benign monoclonal gammopathy
Macroglobulinaemia
Lymphoma
Chronic lymphocytic leukaemia
Chronic cold haemaglutin disease

Platelet function: reduced

Uraemia
Myeloproliferative disease
Leukaemia
Dysproteinaemias

Poikilocytosis: variation in shape

Iron deficiency
Intravascular haemolysis
Bone marrow fibrosis (teardrop cells)

Polycythaemia

Reduced plasma volume (Gaisbock's syndrome)
Polycythaemia rubra vera
Hypoxia
Renal tumour
Adult polycystic kidney disease
Phaeochromocytoma
Cushing's disease

Post-splenectomy: blood film

Howell Jolly bodies
Target cells
Pappenheimer bodies
Heinz bodies

Purpura

Infection
Connective tissue disease
Hereditary haemorrhagic telangiectasia
Scurvy
Amyloid
Steroid therapy

Sickle crisis

Thrombosis
Aplastic crisis
Haemolysis
Sequestration

Sideroblastic anaemia

Anti-tuberculous drugs
Chloramphenicol
Alcohol
Lead poisoning
Myelodysplastic syndrome
Coeliac disease
Rheumatoid arthritis
Carcinoma
X-linked

Target cells

Haemoglobin C disease
Sickle cell anaemia
Iron deficiency
Liver disease
Post-splenectomy
Thalassaemia
Lecithin cholesterol acyl transferase deficiency

Teardrop cell

Bone marrow fibrosis
Thalassaemia

Thrombocytopenia

Reduced production
Bone marrow failure
Metabolic disease
Aplasia of megakaryocyte precursors
Increased breakdown
Autoimmune
Abnormal platelet structure
Sepsis
Drugs
Increased loss
Bleeding
Splenomegaly

Thrombocytosis

Post-splenectomy
Polycythaemia rubra vera
Myelosclerosis
GI bleed
Inflammatory response

Thrombophilia

Protein C/S deficiency
Paroxysmal nocturnal haemoglobinuria
Polycythaemia
Waldenström's macroglobulinaemia
Thrombocythaemia
Systemic lupus erythematosus
Antiphospholipid antibody syndrome
Hyperosmolar non-ketotic coma
Factor V Leiden deficiency
Behcet's syndrome
Homocystinaemia
Malignancy

Tumours and polycythaemia

Renal carcinoma
Cerebellar haemangioblastoma
Hepatoma
Fibroids
Adrenal carcinoma
Wilms' tumour

Cardiology

Aortic dissection

Hypertension
Marfan's syndrome
Ehlers-Danlos syndrome
Coarctation of the aorta
Pregnancy
Trauma

Aortic regurgitation: associations

Hypertension
Marfan's syndrome
Relapsing polychondritis
Syphilis
Ankylosing spondylitis
Rheumatoid arthritis

Aortic stenosis

Congenital
Bicuspid aortic valve
Rheumatic fever
Calcified aortic valve
Infective endocarditis
Supra-valvular stenosis

Atrial fibrillation

Myocardial ischaemia
Thyrotoxicosis
Idiopathic
Sepsis
Wolff Parkinson White syndrome
Alcohol
Dilated left atrium
Sino-atrial disease

Coarctation of the aorta: associations

Bicuspid aortic valve
Turner's syndrome
Berry aneurysm
Ventriculo-septal defect
Patent ductus arteriosus

Complete heart block

Drugs
Digoxin
Verapamil
β-blockers
Infection
Rheumatic fever
Diphtheria
Lyme disease
Myocardial ischaemia
Conduction fibrosis
Metabolic abnormalities
Dystrophia myotonica

Cor pulmonale

Chronic lung disease
Multiple pulmonary emboli
Thoracic wall deformity
Neuromuscular disease
Obesity
Central hypoventilation

Cyanotic heart disease: complications

Cerebral abscess
Iron deficiency
Gout
Polycythaemia
Renal failure
Arthritis
Haemoptysis
Infective endocarditis
Arrhythmias

Dilated cardiomyopathy

Haemochromatosis
Sarcoidosis
Friedreich's ataxia
Duchenne's muscular dystrophy
Alcohol
Amyloidosis
Thyrotoxicosis
Viral myocarditis
Thiamine deficiency
Acromegaly
Chemotherapy
Persistent tachycardia
Post-partum
Idiopathic

Electrocardiogram changes: metabolic

Hypokalaemia
Prolonged PR interval
ST depression
Flattened T waves
U waves
Prolonged QT interval
Hyperkalaemia
Tented T wave
Wide QRS complex
Flat P wave
Reduced R wave amplitude
Hypothermia
J waves
Bradycardia
Atrial fibrillation
Muscle tremor
Prolonged QT interval

Heart failure

Ischaemic heart disease
Cardiomyopathies
Valvular disease
Myocardial fibrosis
Pericardial disease
High output

Hypertension in young person

Endocrine
Hyperaldosteronism
Phaeochromocytoma
Acromegaly
Cushing's syndrome
Primary hyperparathyroidism
Cardiovascular
Renal arterial disease
Coarctation of the aorta
Pre-eclampsia
Pregnancy
Any renal pathology

Left axis deviation

Left anterior hemiblock
Atrio-septal defect (ostium primum)
Wolff Parkinson White syndrome
Pacing wire *in situ*
Myotonic dystrophy
Ventricular tachycardia
Inferior myocardial infarction

Left bundle branch block

Aortic stenosis
Left ventricular hypertrophy
Myocardial infarction
Cardiomyopathy
Conduction system fibrosis

Mitral regurgitation

Infective endocarditis
Rheumatic fever
Floppy mitral valve
Atrio-septal defect
Marfan's syndrome
Cardiomyopathy
Ischaemic heart disease

Myocardial infarction: complications

Arrhythmias
Cardiac failure
Pericarditis
Cardiac rupture
Thromboembolism
Ventricular aneurysm
Papillary muscle rupture
Ventriculoseptal defect
Cardiogenic shock

Pericardial effusion

Viral
Tuberculosis
Bacterial
Neoplastic
Connective tissue disease
Dressler's syndrome
Trauma

Positive R wave in V1

Wolff Parkinson White syndrome type A
True posterior myocardial infarction
Dextrocardia
Right bundle branch block
Duchenne's muscular dystrophy
Right ventricular hypertrophy

PR interval: prolonged

Lyme disease
Tricyclic antidepressants
Atrio-septal defect
Cardiomyopathy
Hypokalaemia
Rheumatic fever

PR interval: short

Wolff Parkinson White syndrome
Lown-Ganong-Levine syndrome
Hypertrophic obstructive cardiomyopathy
Duchenne's muscular dystrophy

Pulmonary hypertension

Primary
Secondary
Hypoxia
Raised left atrial pressure
Pulmonary embolus
Collagen vascular disease
Slimming drugs
Cirrhosis
Sickle cell disease

Pulse pressure: narrow

Aortic stenosis
Constrictive pericarditis
Pericardial effusion
Shock

Pulse pressure: wide

Aortic regurgitation
Patent ductus arteriosus
Thyrotoxicosis
Sepsis
Pregnancy
High output cardiac failure

Pulsus paradoxus

Asthma
Constrictive pericarditis
Cardiac tamponade
Cardiomyopathy

QT interval: increased

Drugs
Amiodarone
Sotalol
Phenothiazines
Tricyclic antidepressants
Terfenadine
Erythromycin
Metabolic disturbance
Hypokalaemia
Hypomagnesaemia
Hypothyroidism
Bradycardia
Congenital
Roman-Ward syndrome
Jervell-Lange-Nielson syndrome

Right axis deviation

Left posterior hemiblock
Atrio-septal defect (ostium secundum)
Right ventricular hypertrophy
Pulmonary stenosis
Fallot's tetralogy

Cardiology

Right bundle branch block

Congenital
Atrio-septal defect
Fallot's tetralogy
Acquired
Ischaemic heart disease
Cardiomyopathy
Myocarditis
Conduction system fibrosis
Pulmonary
Cor pulmonale
Pulmonary embolus

Sinus bradycardia

Hypothyroidism
Hypothermia
Drugs
Athletes
Raised intracranial pressure
Sino-atrial disease

Superior vena cava obstruction

Carcinoma of bronchus
Lymphoma
Thyroid mass
Teratoma
Thoracic aortic aneurysm
Fibrosing mediastinitis

Tricuspid regurgitation

Functional
Carcinoid syndrome
Infective endocarditis
Rheumatic fever
Cirrhosis
Endomyocardial fibrosis

Ventricular fibrillation

Myocardial ischaemia
Ventricular tachycardia
Electric shock
Wolff Parkinson White syndrome
Severe electrolyte disturbance
Left ventricular hypertrophy
Prolonged QT interval

Infectious disease/HIV

AIDS-defining illness

Cryptococcal infection
Kaposi's sarcoma <60 years old
Progressive multifocal leucoencephalopathy
Toxoplasmosis
Oesophageal candidiasis
Disseminated cytomegalovirus

Bleeding tendency

Leptospirosis
Ebola virus
Yellow fever

Cervical lymphadenopathy (bilateral)

Cytomegalovirus
Epstein Barr virus
HIV
Lymphoma
Tuberculosis
Phenytoin

Congenital cytomegalovirus

Choroidoretinitis
Purpura
Recurrent respiratory tract infections
Hepatosplenomegaly
Microcephaly
Deafness
Cerebral calcification

Congenital infections

Toxoplasmosis
Syphilis
Rubella
Cytomegalovirus
Herpes

DNA virus

Herpes
Hepatitis B
Pox
Adenovirus
Epstein Barr virus
Cytomegalovirus
Varicella Zoster virus

Duckett Jones criteria

Major
Carditis
Polyarthritis
Sydenham's chorea
Erythema marginatum
Subcutaneous nodules
Minor
Arthralgia
Fever
Raised ESR/CRP
Prolonged PR interval

Epstein Barr Virus: complications

Meningitis
Arthritis
Myocarditis
Agranulocytosis
Glomerulonephritis
Haemolysis
Burkitt's lymphoma
Nasopharyngeal carcinoma

Exotoxins

Streptococcus
E. coli
Vibrio cholera
Clostridium
Shigella

Fever in traveller

Short incubation
Hepatitis A
Malaria
Typhoid
Leptospirosis
Haemorrhagic fevers
Dengue
Long incubation
Malaria
Typhoid
Leishmaniasis
Tuberculosis
Brucellosis
Amoebic abscess

Food poisoning

Bacillus cereus
Vibrio parahaemolyticus
Clostridium perfringens
Salmonella
Shigella
Campylobacter

Gonorrhoea: systemic complications

Tenosynovitis
Pustular rash
Meningitis
Endocarditis
Perihepatitis

HIV: central nervous system

Toxoplasmosis
Cryptococcal meningitis
Progressive multifocal leucoencephalopathy
Cytomegalovirus
HIV encephalopathy
Pyogenic abscess

HIV: diarrhoea

Cryptosporidium
Giardia
Entamoeba histolytica
Mycobacterium avium intracellulare
Idiopathic

HIV: oral problems

Candida albicans
Candida creusi
Oral hairy leukoplakia
Gingivitis

HIV: retinal problems

Cytomegalovirus retinitis
Toxoplasmosis
Choroidoretinitis
Fungal infection
Bacterial infection

HIV treatment

Nucleoside analogues
Zidovudine
ddl
ddC
Lamivudine
Non-nucleoside analogues
Nevirapine
Protease inhibitors
Saquinavir

Hyperpyrexia

Infection
Heat stroke
Neuroleptic malignant syndrome
Malignant hyperthermia
Ecstasy
Cocaine
Amphetamines

Jaundice in the tropics

Hepatitis
Malaria
Typhoid
Yellow fever
Leptospirosis
G6PD and anti-malarials
Thalassaemia
Sickle cell disease

Kawasaki's disease

Fever
Conjunctivitis
Mucous membrane involvement
Rash
Desquamation of extremities
Cervical lymphadenopathy

Live vaccines

Polio
Small pox
Yellow fever
Rubella
Tuberculosis

Lymphocytic meningitis

Mycoplasma
Cryptococcal meningitis
Brucellosis
Lyme disease
Epstein Barr virus
Leptospirosis

Malaise and HIV (nil focal)

Mycobacterium
Cytomegalovirus
Toxoplasma
Pneumocystis carinii
Cryptococcus
Histoplasmosis
Coccidiomycosis
Legionella
Drug adverse effects
Lymphoma
Kaposi's sarcoma

Meningitis: age distribution

Neonatal
E. coli
Group B streptococcus
Listeria
Pre-school
Haemophilus influenzae
Neisseria meningitides
Adults
Neisseria meningitides
Streptococcus pneumoniae

Pancytopenia and HIV

Zidovudine
Co-trimoxazole
HIV marrow disease
Lymphoma
Mycobacterial marrow infiltration
Epstein Barr virus

Pneumocystis carinii: treatment

Co-trimoxazole
Nebulised pentamidine
Clindamycin
Primaquine
Dapsone

Positive VDRL

Treponemal infection
Yaws
Leptospirosis
Epstein Barr virus
Mycoplasma
Bacterial endocarditis
Autoimmune
Systemic lupus erythematosus
Sjögren's syndrome
Hashimoto's disease

Pyrexia of unknown origin

Infective
Pyogenic abscess
Tuberculosis
Endocarditis
Urinary tract infection
Viral infection
Amoebic abscess
Brucellosis
Non-infective
Malignancy
Lymphoma
Leukaemia
Connective tissue disease

RNA virus

Enterovirus
Paramyxovirus
Rubella
Hepatitis A
Measles
Influenza

Streptococcal pneumonia in young person

Hypogammaglobulinaemia
Hyposplenism
Alcohol
HIV
Systemic lupus erythematosus

Tick-borne infection

Rickettsia
Flavivirus infection
Lyme disease
Relapsing fever
Rocky Mountain fever
Q fever

Tropical eosinophilia

Hookworm
Ascaris
Strongyloides
Schistosomiasis
Filariasis
Trichinosis

Typhoid: complications

Bowel perforation
Neuropsychiatric disease
Pneumonia
Nephritis
Hepatitis
Rose spots
Bradycardia

Neurology

Abdominal pain and neuropathy

Acute intermittent porphyria
Diabetes mellitus
Lead poisoning
Guillain Barré syndrome
Carcinomatosis

Absent reflexes with up-going plantars

Anterior horn cell disease
Friedreich's ataxia
Tabes dorsalis
Subacute combined degeneration of the cord
Spinal shock
Pellagra
Conus medullaris lesion

Autonomic neuropathy

Diabetes mellitus
Sarcoidosis
Amyloidosis
Shy-Drager syndrome
Viral infection
Renal failure
Chagas' disease
Tetanus
Alcohol
B12 deficiency
Guillain Barré syndrome

Axonal changes on electromyogram

Hereditary sensori-motor neuropathy type 1
Toxins/drugs
Polio
Motor neurone disease
Ischaemia
Uraemia
Porphyria

Benign intracranial hypertension

Drugs
Dural sinus thrombosis
Pregnancy
Hypoparathyroidism
Idiopathic

Berry aneurysm

Adult polycystic kidney disease
Marfan's syndrome
Ehlers-Danlos syndrome
Pseudoxanthoma elasticum
Cervical artery dissection
Fibromuscular dysplasia
Hereditary haemorrhagic telangiectasia
Klinefelter's syndrome

Bilateral facial nerve palsy

Guillain Barré syndrome
Sarcoidosis
Lyme disease
Myopathy
Anterior horn cell disease
HIV conversion

Bilateral ptosis

Myasthenia gravis
Myotonic dystrophy
Congenital
Bilateral Horner's syndrome
Bilateral third nerve palsy
Kearns-Sayre syndrome

Bulbar palsy

Guillain Barré syndrome
Anterior horn cell disease
Poliomyelitis
Syringobulbia

Carpal tunnel syndrome

Pregnancy
Hypothyroidism
Acromegaly
Rheumatoid arthritis
Oral contraceptive pill
Idiopathic
Diabetes mellitus
Amyloid

Cerebellar signs

Disdiadokinesis
Ataxia
Nystagmus
Intention tremor
Staccato speech
Hypotonia
DANISH

Cerebellopontine angle lesions

Acoustic neuroma
Meningioma
Basilar artery aneurysm
Cholesteatoma
Haemangioblastoma

Cerebrospinal fluid: raised protein with normal cells

Guillain Barré syndrome
Acoustic neuroma
Froin's syndrome (spinal cord block)
Subacute sclerosing panencephalitis
Lead poisoning

Chorea

Huntington's disease
Sydenham's chorea
Systemic lupus erythematosus
Wilson's disease
Pregnancy
Thyrotoxicosis
Oral contraceptive pill
Polycythaemia
Hypoparathyroidism

Cortical vein thrombosis

Local sepsis
Surgery
Tumour invading sinus
Venous catheterization
Dehydration
Oral contraceptive pill
Pregnancy
Thrombophilia

Delayed visual evoked potential

Demyelination
Friedreich's ataxia
B12 deficiency
Optic nerve compression
Glaucoma

Demyelinating changes on electromyogram

Multiple sclerosis
Lead poisoning
Diphtheria
Guillain Barré syndrome
Diabetes mellitus
Leprosy
Hereditary sensori-motor neuropathy type 2

Dystonia

Drugs
Idiopathic
Wilson's disease
Mitochondrial disease
Spinocerebellar degeneration

Dystrophia myotonica: complications

Diabetes mellitus
Testicular atrophy
Conduction defect
Cardiomyopathy
Cataracts
Anaesthetic risk
Thyroid dysfunction

Epilepsy

Idiopathic
Vascular
Congenital
Tumour
Infection
Alcohol
Trauma

Hypothyroidism: neurological sequelae

Carpal tunnel
Slow relaxing reflexes
Pendred's syndrome (deafness)
Cerebellar ataxia
Proximal myopathy
Myxoedema madness
Dementia

Hypotonia

Lower motor neurone lesion
Cerebellar disease
Tabes dorsalis
Spinal shock

Intracerebral calcification

Sturge-Weber-Dimitri syndrome (parallel lines on SXR)
Tuberous sclerosis
Congenital toxoplasma
Cytomegalovirus
Tuberculosis
Cysticercosis
Angioma
Haematoma
Craniopharyngioma
Pinealoma

Lymphocytes in cerebrospinal fluid

Tuberculosis
Viral meningitis/encephalitis
Fungal meningitis
Meningovascular syphilis
Toxoplasmosis
Neurosarcoidosis
Lymphoma
Central nervous system inflammatory disease

Mitochondrial cytopathies

Myoclonic epilepsy with ragged red fibres
MELAS syndrome
Leber's optic atrophy
Kearns-Sayre syndrome

Mononeuritis multiplex

Diabetes mellitus
Sarcoidosis
Rheumatoid arthritis
Carcinomatosis
Systemic lupus erythematosus
Leprosy
HIV
Polyarteritis nodosa
Churg-Strauss syndrome
Cryoglobulinaemia

Motor neuropathy

Polio
Guillain Barré syndrome
Acute intermittent porphyria
Lead poisoning

Multiple sclerosis: good prognostic features

Young age of onset
Optic neuritis
No cerebellar signs
Complete recovery

Myoclonus

Hereditary
Creutzfeldt-Jakob disease
Alzheimer's disease
Tay Sach's disease
Gaucher's disease
Acute metabolic encephalopathy

Nerve thickening

Tuberculous leprosy
Amyloid
Sarcoidosis
Neurofibromatosis
Acromegaly
Refsum's disease
Hereditary sensori-motor neuropathy type 1

Neurofibromatosis: associations

Acoustic neuroma
Schwannoma
Optic glioma
Meningioma
Multiple endocrine neoplasia type 2
Café au lait patches
Lung fibrosis
Restrictive cardiomyopathy

Parkinsonism

Parkinson's disease
Drug induced
Carbon monoxide
MPTP
Encephalitis

Parkinson's plus

Multiple system atrophy
Progressive supranuclear palsy
Basal ganglia calcification
Corticobasal degeneration

Periodic electroencephalogram

Subacute sclerosing panencephalitis
Herpes encephalitis
Hepatic coma
Creutzfeldt-Jakob disease
Carbon monoxide poisoning (slow EEG)
Petit mal (3:1 spike and wave)

Pes cavus

Spina bifida
Polio
Friedreich's ataxia
Hereditary sensori-motor neuropathy
Syringomyelia
Homocysteinuria

Pseudobulbar palsy

Cerebrovascular disease
Demyelination
Anterior horn cell disease

Ptosis

Neurogenic
3rd nerve palsy
Horner's syndrome
Myogenic
Congenital
Myasthenia gravis
Dystrophia myotonia
Ocular myopathy

Small muscle wasting of hands

T1
Motor neurone disease
Syringomyelia
Spinal cord compression
Syphilis
Polio
Root lesion
Cervical spondylosis
Neurofibroma
Brachial plexus
Cervical rib
Pancoast's tumour
Klumpke's palsy
Peripheral
Ulnar/median nerve palsy
Rheumatoid arthritis

Spastic paraparesis

Demyelination
Cord compression
Anterior horn cell disease
Friedreich's ataxia
Syringomyelia
Anterior spinal artery thrombosis
Subacute combined degeneration of the cord
Parasaggital meningioma
Taboparesis
Transverse myelitis
HIV myelitis
Mycoplasma
Hereditary spastic paraparesis
Tropical spastic paraparesis

Third nerve palsy

Mononeuritis multiplex
Posterior communicating aneurysm
Demyelination
Ischaemia in midbrain
Cavernous sinus syndromes

Tremor

Resting
Parkinsonism
Extrapyramidal disease
Postural
Benign essential tremor
Thyrotoxicosis
Anxiety
Sympathomimetic drugs
Intention
Cerebellar disease
Brain stem disease

Wernicke's encephalopathy

Vitamin B1 deficiency
Alcohol
Carcinoma of the stomach
Malabsorption
Haemodialysis
Hyperemesis gravidarum
Anorexia nervosa

Therapeutics

Alopecia

Valproate
Heparin
Warfarin
Vitamin A toxicity
Methotrexate
Cytotoxics
Atenolol
Sulphasalazine

Benign intracranial hypertension

Oral contraceptive pill
Vitamin A deficiency
Retinoids
Tetracyclines
Steroids
Nitrofurantoin

Breast feeding: drugs to avoid

Lithium
Tetracyclines
Aspirin
Benzodiazepines
Isotretinoin

Cataracts

Amiodarone
Chloroquine
Steroids

Cholestasis

Sulphonamides
Tricyclic antidepressants
Oral contraceptive pill
Phenothiazines
Non-steroidal anti-inflammatory drugs
Antibiotics e.g. penicillin, erythromycin
Sulphonylureas
Anti-tuberculous drugs
Carbimazole

Convulsions

Anti-histamines
Mefenamic acid
Tricyclic antidepressants
Oral hypoglycaemics
Lignocaine
Phenothiazines

Diabetogenic drugs

Steroids
Thiazides
Loop diuretics

Digoxin toxicity

Extracardiac
Anorexia
Fatigue
Diarrhoea
Xanthopsia
Cardiac
Ventricular ectopics
Ventricular bigeminy
Ventricular tachycardia
Complete heart block
Reverse tick

Drugs causing Coomb's positive haemolysis

Rifampicin
Isoniazid
Benzylpenicillin
Septrin
Methyldopa
Quinine

Drugs causing erythema multiforme

Sulphonamides
Salicylates
Barbiturates
Penicillins
Sulphonylureas

Drug-induced lupus

Chlorpromazine
Hydralazine
Isoniazid
Procainamide
Phenytoin
Beta blockers

Enzyme inducers

Phenytoin
Carbamazepine
Barbiturates
Rifampicin
Alcohol
Sulphonylureas
PCBRAS

Enzyme inhibitors

Omeprazole
Disulfiram
Ethanol
Valproate
Cimetidine, ciprofloxacin
Erythromycin
Sulphonylureas
ODEVICES

Goitre

Lithium
Carbimazole
Iodine
Phenylbutazone

Gynaecomastia

Digoxin
Spironolactone
Methyldopa
Cimetidine
Oestrogens
Anti-androgens

Haemodialysis in toxicity

Salicylates
Lithium
Theophyllines
Barbiturates
Antifreeze/methanol/ethanol

Hepatitis

Methotrexate
Isoniazid
Amiodarone
Phenelzine
Halothane
Methyldopa
Statins
Non-steroidal anti-inflammatory drugs
Rifampicin
Ketoconazole

Hirsutism

Phenytoin
Diazoxide
Minoxidil
Cyclosporin A
Steroids
Progestogens

Hypertension

Steroids
Oral contraceptive pill
DDAVP
Monoamine oxidase inhibitors
Carbenoxolone

Lead poisoning: side effects

Motor neuropathy
Gingivitis
Basophilic stippling on blood film
Cerebral oedema
Constipation

Lichen planus

Methyldopa
Penicillamine
Sulphonamides
Sulphonylureas
Thiazide diuretics

Lung fibrosis

Bleiomycin
Busulphan
Nitrofurantoin
Amiodarone
Methotrexate

Macrocytosis

Methotrexate
Azathioprine
Phenytoin
Anti-retrovirals

Neutropenia

Carbimazole
Anticonvulsants
Phenothiazines
Chloramphenicol
Sulphonamides
Cytotoxics

Optic neuritis

Ethambutol
Streptomycin
Isoniazid

Oxidising drugs

Dapsone
Sulphonamides
Nitrofurantoin
Antimalarials
Ciprofloxacin

Painful myopathy

Diamorphine
Barbiturates
Diazepam
Carbenoxolone
Amphotericin
Isoniazid

Peripheral neuropathy

Metronidazole
Isoniazid
Nitrofurantoin
Vincristine/vinblastine
Cisplatinum
Amiodarone
Phenytoin

Photosensitivity

Thiazides
Tetracyclines
Amiodarone
Tricyclic antidepressants
Griseofulvin

Pigmentation

Minocycline
Antimalarials
Phenothiazines
Busulphan

Retroperitoneal fibrosis

Methysergide
Methyldopa
Bromocriptine

Sulphasalazine: side effects

Neutropenia
Liver granulomas
Stevens-Johnson syndrome
Eosinophilic pneumonia
Haemolysis
Lung fibrosis
Alopecia

Syndrome of inappropriate ADH

Chlorpropamide
Chlorpromazine
Carbamazepine
Opiates
Tricyclic antidepressants
Cytotoxics
Rifampicin

Thrombocytopenia

Quinine
Co-trimoxazole
Heparin
Non-steroidal anti-inflammatory drugs
Thiazides
Gold
Chloramphenicol

Zero order kinetics

Alcohol
Phenytoin
Hydralazine
Disulfiram

Dermatology

Acanthosis nigricans

Carcinoma
Stomach
Oesophagus
Colon
Bladder
Kidney
Miscellaneous
Insulin resistance
Acromegaly
Prader-Willi syndrome
Steroids

Bullous skin lesions

Pemphigus
Pemphigoid
Dermatitis herpetiformis
Erythema multiforme
Porphyria
Snake/insect bites

Café au lait patches: associations

Neurofibromatosis
Subacute bacterial endocarditis
Thyrotoxicosis
Albright's syndrome
Tuberous sclerosis
Fibrous dysplasia

Complement deposition and skin

Pemphigus
Pemphigoid
Systemic lupus erythematosus
Dermatitis herpetiformis

Cutaneous markers of malignancy

Acanthosis nigricans
Dermatomyositis
Herpes zoster
Necrolytic migratory erythema

Desquamating rash

Scarlet fever
Toxic shock syndrome
Kawasaki's disease
Drug reaction

Eruptive xanthomata

Hyperlipidaemia
Diabetes
Liver disease
Nephrotic syndrome
Myxoedema
Chronic pancreatitis

Erythema multiforme

Idiopathic
Streptococcus
Mycoplasma
Histoplasmosis
HIV
Systemic lupus erythematosus
Carcinoma
Drugs

Erythema nodosum

Crohn's disease
Ulcerative colitis
Tuberculosis
Behcet's syndrome
Atypical pneumonia
Drugs e.g. sulphonamides/oral contraceptives
Sarcoidosis
Other infections e.g. measles/pertussis/streptococcus
Idiopathic
Leprosy/lymphogranuloma venereum
Leukaemia
CUTBADSOIL

Erythroderma

Eczema
Psoriasis
Lymphoma
Sézary syndrome
Drugs

Hyperhydrosis

Sepsis
Thyrotoxicosis
Lymphoma
Malignancy
Hypoglycaemia
Acromegaly
Gustatory sweating
Sympathetic dysfunction

Hyperkeratosis (palmoplantar)

Secondary syphilis
Keratoderma blennorrhagicum
Hypovitaminosis A
Arsenic

Hypertrichosis

General
Anorexia nervosa
Malnutrition
Drugs
Androgenisation
Local
Spina bifida
Pigmented naevus
Lichen simplex

Koebner's phenomenon

Psoriasis
Lichen planus
Molluscum contagiosum
Vitiligo
Viral warts

Leukoplakia

Candida
HIV
Trauma
Treponemal disease

Livedo reticularis

Cryoglobulinaemia
Systemic lupus erythematosus
Cholesterol embolus

Onycholysis

Trauma
Psoriasis
Eczema
Graves' disease
Tetracyclines

Orogenital ulceration

Behcet's disease
Reiter's syndrome
Pemphigus
Crohn's disease
Syphilis
Herpes simplex
Erythema multiforme
Strachan's syndrome

Palmar erythema

Liver disease
Pregnancy
Thyrotoxicosis
Chronic leukaemia

Pigmentation

Haemochromatosis
Addison's disease
Nelson's syndrome
Peutz-Jegher's syndrome
Urticaria pigmentosa
Chloasma of pregnancy
Café au lait patches
Fungal infection
Drugs
Anti-malarials
Tetracyclines

Pruritis

Malignancy
Uraemia
Diabetes
Myxoedema
Thyrotoxicosis
Biliary obstruction
Iron deficiency
Polycythaemia

Pyoderma gangrenosum

Inflammatory bowel disease
Rheumatoid arthritis
Wegener's granulomatosis
Myeloma
Lymphoma
Idiopathic

Scarring alopecia

Systemic lupus erythematosus
Lichen planus
Lupus vulgaris
Trauma
Burns

Subcutaneous calcification

CREST syndrome
Dermatomyositis
Cysticercosis
Loa loa
Trichinella

Vitiligo: associations

Addison's disease
Diabetes mellitus
Hypoparathyroidism
Ovarian failure
Renal tubular acidosis
Chronic active hepatitis
Autoimmune thyroid disease

Ophthalmology

Angioid streaks

Pseudoxanthoma elasticum
Ehlers-Danlos syndrome
Sickle cell anaemia
Paget's disease
Acromegaly
Hypercalcaemia
Lead poisoning

Blue sclerae

Marfan's syndrome
Ehlers-Danlos syndrome
Pseudoxanthoma elasticum
Osteogenesis imperfecta

Cherry-red spot on macula

Early central retinal artery occlusion
Niemann-Pick disease
Tay-Sach's disease
Carbon monoxide poisoning
Sialidosis

Choroidoretinitis

Idiopathic
Toxoplasmosis
Congenital CMV
Congenital rubella
Diabetes
Sarcoidosis

Congenital cataracts

Dystrophia myotonica
Galactosaemia
Down syndrome
Refsum's disease
Lawrence-Moon-Biedle syndrome
Congenital hypothyroidism
Rubella

Diabetic retinopathy

Background
Dot/blot haemorrhages
Microaneurysms
Hard exudates
Preproliferative
Background + soft exudates
Proliferative
Proproliferative + new vessels
Maculopathy

Hypertensive retinopathy

Grade 1
Silver wiring
Grade 2
AV nipping
Grade 3
Flame haemorrhages
Soft exudates
Grade 4
Papilloedema

Iritis

Infection
Rheumatoid
Immune
Trauma
Idiopathic
Sarcoidosis
IRITIS

Optic atrophy

Hereditary
Leber's congenital amaurosis
Friedreich's ataxia
DIDMOAD
Acquired
Glaucoma
Retinal artery occlusion
Demyelination
Diabetes
Tobacco/alcohol amblyopia
Chronic papilloedema

Papilloedema

Raised intracranial pressure
Benign intracranial hypertension
Retinal vein thrombosis
Hypoparathyroidism
Lead poisoning
Hypercapnia
Vitamin A toxicity

Proliferative retinopathy

Diabetes mellitus
Retinal vein thrombosis
Sickle cell anaemia
Systemic lupus erythematosus
Eales' syndrome

Pupillary abnormalities

Argyll Robertson pupil
Gunn's pupil
Holmes-Adie syndrome

Relative afferent papillary defect

Central retinal artery occlusion
Optic neuritis
Optic nerve compression
Retinal detachment
Unilateral glaucoma

Retinal artery occlusion

Atheroma
Thromboembolism
Vasculitis
Sickle cell disease

Retinal vein thrombosis

Hypertension
Diabetes mellitus
Hyperlipidaemia
Thrombophilia
Vasculitis
Glaucoma

Retinitis pigmentosa

Refsum's disease
Abetalipoproteinaemia
Friedreich's ataxia
Lawrence-Moon-Biedle syndrome
Kearns-Sayre syndrome
Usher's syndrome
Idiopathic
Hallervorden-Spatz disease

Roth's spots

Infective endocarditis
Systemic lupus erythematosus
Polyarteritis nodosa

Rubeosis iris

Proliferative retinopathy
Central retinal vein occlusion
Carotid ischaemia
Chronic retinal detachment
Intraocular tumour

Sacroiliitis

Reiter's disease
Ankylosing spondylitis
Psoriasis
Enteropathic

Scleromalacia perforans

Rheumatoid arthritis
Ankylosing spondylitis
Herpes zoster
Wegener's granulomatosis
Polyarteritis nodosa
Gout

Tunnel vision

Retinitis pigmentosa
Papilloedema
Glaucoma
Tabes
Migraine
Hysteria
Choroidoretinitis

Unilateral exophthalmos

Grave's disease
Tumour/granuloma
Cavernous sinus thrombosis
Caroticocavernous fistula
Cellulitis
Periostitis

Uveitis

Sarcoidosis
Vasculitis
HIV
Tuberculosis
Crohn's disease
Seronegative arthropathy

Xanthomata

Familial hypercholesterolaemia
Diabetes mellitus
Hypothyroidism
Nephrotic syndrome
Primary biliary cirrhosis

Respiratory

Bilateral hilar lymphadenopathy

Sarcoidosis
Tuberculosis
Lymphoma
Bronchial carcinoma
Histoplasma
Silicosis

Bronchiectasis

Congenital immune deficiency
Ciliary abnormalities
Cystic fibrosis
Kartagener's syndrome
Infection
Tuberculosis
Whooping cough
Measles
Inflammation
Inflammatory bowel disease
Rheumatoid arthritis
Vasculitis

Calcification of lung fields

Asbestos exposure
Histoplasmosis
Tuberculosis
Varicella Zoster virus pneumonia
Sarcoidosis
Silicosis

Cannon ball lesions

Sarcoma
Teratoma
Renal carcinoma

Cavitating lung lesion

Abscess
Carcinoma
Tuberculosis
Wegener's granulomatosis
Fungal infection
Infarction
Hydatid cysts

Fibrosis with normal lung volume

Tuberous sclerosis
Histiocytosis X
Lymphangiomyomatosis
Neurofibromatosis

Granulomatous lung disease

Churg-Strauss syndrome
Sarcoidosis
Wegener's granulomatosis
Histiocytosis X
Infective

Honeycomb lung

Histiocytosis X
Neurofibromatosis
Tuberous sclerosis
Lymphangiomyomatosis

Lung abscess

Staphylococcus aureus
Klebsiella
Tuberculosis
Bacteroides
Actinomycoses
Histoplasmosis
Coccidiomycosis
Aspergillus
Amoebic abscess

Lung fibrosis

Cryptogenic fibrosing alveolitis
Systemic sclerosis
Systemic lupus erythematosus
Ankylosing spondylitis
Sjögren's syndrome
Polymyositis
Drugs
Radiotherapy
Rheumatoid arthritis
Extrinsic allergic alveolitis
Asbestosis
Inorganic chemical exposure

Mediastinal tumours

Anterior
Lymphoma
Thymoma
Thyroid mass
Dermoid cyst
Pericardial cyst
Ascending aortic aneurysm
Teratoma
Posterior
Ganglioneuroma
Paravertebral mass
Descending aortic aneurysm

Miliary shadowing on CXR

Miliary tuberculosis
Sarcoidosis
Pneumoconiosis
Haemosiderosis
Lymphangitis carcinomatosis
Silicosis

Pleural effusion

Transudate
Congestive cardiac failure
Cirrhosis
Nephrotic syndrome
Hypothyroidism
Exudate
Malignancy
Infection
Vasculitis
Pulmonary infarction
Meig's syndrome
Dressler's syndrome
Yellow nail syndrome

Pulmonary eosinophilia

Eosinophilic pneumonia
Asthma
Tropical infection
Allergic bronchopulmonary aspergillosis
Churg-Strauss syndrome
Wegener's granulomatosis

Pulmono-renal syndromes

Goodpasture's syndrome
Polyarteritis nodosa
Wegener's granulomatosis
Bronchial Ca with membranous glomerulonephritis
Legionella
Mycoplasma

Rheumatoid arthritis and lung problems

Pleural effusion
Nodules
Fibrosing alveolitis
Obliterative bronchiolitis
Vasculitis
Caplan's syndrome

Rib notching

Coarctation of the aorta
Neurofibromatosis
Hypertrophy of nerves
Inferior vena cava obstruction
Blalock shunt
Congenital

Scoliosis

Idiopathic
Surgery
Neuromuscular
Poliomyelitis
Friedreich's ataxia
Syringomyelia
Duchenne's muscular dystrophy
Connective tissue disease
Marfan's syndrome
Osteogenesis imperfecta

Sickle cell and lung problems

Pneumococcal pneumonia
Pulmonary infarction
Lung sequestration
Interstitial fibrosis
Cor pulmonale

Solitary lesion on CXR

Bronchial carcinoma
Bronchial adenoma
Metastasis
Granuloma
Fibroma
Haematoma
Hydatid cyst

Systemic lupus erythematosus and lung

Shrinking lung
Pneumonitis
Pleurisy
Pulmonary embolus
Immunosuppressant related infections
Drug-induced fibrosis

Transfer factor (KCO): raised

Pulmonary haemorrhage
Asthma
Polycythaemia
Pneumonectomy
Left to right shunt

Transfer factor (KCO): reduced

Anaemia
Interstitial lung disease
Pulmonary embolus
Arterio-venous malformation

Upper zone fibrosis

Bronchopulmonary aspergillosis
Extrinsic allergic alveolitis
Ankylosing spondylitis
Sarcoidosis
Tuberculosis
BEAST

Rheumatology

Ankylosing spondylitis: associations

Upper zone lung fibrosis
Aortic incompetence
Cardiac defects
Iritis

Anticardiolipin antibody

Medications
Autoimmune diseases
HIV
Infections
Neoplasia
MAIN

Avascular necrosis

Steroids
Scaphoid/neck of femur fracture
Sickle cell
Radiotherapy
Alcohol
Pregnancy
Caisson's disease
Cushing's syndrome
Connective tissue disease
Pancreatitis
Weber-Christian disease
Renal replacement therapy

Behcet's: complications

Orogenital ulceration
Uveitis
Arthritis
Meningo-encephalitis
Thrombophilia
Gastrointestinal problems

Bowing of tibia

Paget's disease
Syphilis
Rickets
Albright's syndrome
Yaws

Chondrocalcinosis

Wilson's disease
Haemochromatosis, hyperparathyroidism
Idiopathic
Pseudogout
Acromegaly
Aging
Diabetes mellitus
Ochronosis
Gout
WHIPADOG

Clubbing

Idiopathic
Respiratory
Bronchial carcinoma
Suppurative lung disease
Lung fibrosis
Abdominal
Inflammatory bowel disease
Cirrhosis
Cardiovascular
Cyanotic heart disease
Infective endocarditis

Dactylitis

Psoriatic arthropathy
Sarcoidosis
Sickle cell disease
Gonococcal infection

Erythrocyte sedimentation rate: elevated

Polymyalgia rheumatica
Temporal arteritis
Myeloma
Waldenström's macroglobulinaemia
Hypernephroma
Vasculitis
Sjögren's syndrome
Malignancy
Viral illness
Tuberculosis
Bacterial sepsis
Idiopathic

Frontal bossing

Thalassaemia
Acromegaly
Hydrocephalus
Achondroplasia
Gorlin's syndrome
Rickets
Paget's disease

HLA-B27: associations

Ankylosing spondylitis
Psoriatic arthropathy
Reiter's syndrome
Reactive arthropathy
Enteropathic arthritis
Behcet's disease

Hypertrophic pulmonary osteoarthropathy

Carcinoma of bronchus
Bronchiectasis
Crohn's disease
Primary biliary cirrhosis
Cyanotic heart disease
Ulcerative colitis
Chronic infections
Mesothelioma
Arterio-venous fistulae
Cirrhosis
Hepatoma
Thymoma
Thalassaemia
Infective endocarditis
Graves' disease

Jaccoud's arthropathy

Systemic lupus erythematosus
Rheumatic fever
Bronchial carcinoma

Marfan's syndrome

Autosomal dominant
Upward lens displacement
Aortic regurgitation
Normal IQ
Inflammatory bowel disease
Cyanotic heart disease
Bacterial endocarditis
Cirrhosis

Myopathy

Polymyositis/dermatomyositis
Endocrine
Acromegaly
Thyroid dysfunction
Hyperparathyroidism
Cushing's syndrome
Addison's disease
Carcinoid syndrome
Hyperaldosteronism
Metabolic
Any electrolyte abnormality
Uraemia
Hepatic failure
Glycogen storage disease
ATP abnormalities
Lipid storage disease

Osteopetrosis

Paget's disease
Fluorosis
Vitamin A toxicity
Oxaluria
Marble bone disease
Angelman's syndrome

Osteoporosis

Endocrine
Thyrotoxicosis
Cushing's syndrome
Hypo-oestrogenism
Hypo-androgenism
Hypopituitarism
Hyperprolactinaemia
Genetic
Osteogenesis imperfecta
Miscellaneous
Drugs
Malnutrition
Malabsorption
Mastocytosis

Psoriatic arthropathy: 5 types

Terminal interphalangeal joints
Rheumatoid arthritis-like
Arthritis mutilans
Asymmetrical oligoarticular
Ankylosing spondylitis

Raynaud's phenomenon

Connective tissue disease

Systemic sclerosis
Systemic lupus erythematosus
Rheumatoid arthritis
Dermatomyositis

Neurogenic

Thoracic outlet syndrome
Carpal tunnel syndrome
Vascular disease
Cold agglutinins
Macroglobulinaemia
Cryoglobulinaemia

Occupational

Reiter's syndrome

Urethritis
Arthritis
Conjunctivitis
Keratoderma blennorrhagicum
Circinate balanitis
Oral ulceration

Rhabdomyolysis

Trauma
Burns
Polymyositis
Ischaemia
Exercise
Convulsions
Alcohol/heroin abuse

Rheumatoid arthritis and anaemia

Non-steroidal anti-inflammatory drugs
Chronic disease
Felty's syndrome
Drugs causing bone marrow suppression
Megaloblastic anaemia
Folate deficiency
Haemolysis
Pernicious anaemia

Rheumatoid arthritis and renal failure

Amyloidosis
Non-steroidal anti-inflammatory drugs
Renal vasculitis

Saddle nose

Wegener's granulomatosis
Trauma
Congenital syphilis
Relapsing polychondritis
Lepromatous leprosy

Scleroderma: antibodies

Antinuclear antibodies (nucleolar)
Anticentromere antibodies
Anti-Scl70

Splinter haemorrhages

Trauma
Infective endocarditis
Vasculitis
Mitral stenosis

Systemic lupus erythematosus: antibodies

Anti-dsDNA
Anti-Sm
Anti-RNP (overlap syndromes)
Anti-Ro
Anti-La
Anticardiolipin

Systemic sclerosis: complications

Raynaud's phenomenon
Sicca syndrome
Oesophageal reflux/stenosis
Intestinal immotility
Pulmonary fibrosis
Myocardial fibrosis

Vasculitis: primary

Large vessel (with granulomas)
Giant cell arteritis
Takayasu's disease
Medium vessel (no granulomas)
Polyarteritis nodosa
Kawasaki's disease
Small vessel (with granulomas)
Wegener's granulomatosis
Churg-Strauss syndrome
Small vessel (no granulomas)
Microscopic polyarteritis nodosa
Henoch-Schönlein purpura

Part B

Acromegaly

Active vs. inactive
Carpal tunnel syndrome
Dilated cardiomyopathy
Hypertension in young person

Addison's disease

Hypercalcaemia
Hyperkalaemia
Hypoglycaemia
Hyponatraemia
Skin pigmentation
Vitiligo: associations

Adult polycystic kidney disease

Berry aneurysms
Congenital renal disease
Enlarged kidney (unilateral)
Polycythaemia
Renal failure with normal/large kidneys
Salt-losing nephritis

Alcohol

Acidosis with raised anion gap
Autonomic neuropathy
Bilateral parotid swelling
Cardiomyopathy
Chronic liver disease
Enzyme inducers
Enzyme inhibitors
Hepatomegaly
Hypercortisolism
Hypoglycaemia
Macrocytosis
Optic atrophy
Osteoporosis
Painful myopathy
Pancreatitis
Raised creatine kinase
Secondary hyperlipidaemia
Sideroblastic anaemia
Wernicke's encephalopathy

Amiodarone

Cataracts
Hypothyroidism
Lung fibrosis
Peripheral neuropathy
Photosensitivity
QT interval: raised
Thyrotoxicosis

Amyloidosis

Autonomic neuropathy
Bilateral parotid swelling
Cardiomyopathy
Hypoadrenalism
Hyposplenism
Macroglossia
Nephrotic syndrome
Nerve thickening
Renal failure with normal sized kidneys
Rheumatoid arthritis and renal failure

Ankylosing spondylitis

Aortic regurgitation
Iritis
Psoriatic arthropathy
Scleromalacia perforans
Upper zone lung fibrosis

Anticonvulsants

Carbamazepine
Syndrome of inappropriate ADH
Phenytoin
Cervical lymphadenopathy
Drug-induced lupus
Enzyme inducers
Gingival hypertrophy
Hirsutism
Macrocytosis
Osteomalacia
Peripheral neuropathy
Valproate
Alopecia
Enzyme inhibitors

Bacterial endocarditis

Café au lait patches: associations
Clubbing: causes
Renal failure and low complement
Roth's spots
Splinter haemorrhages
VDRL: positive

Behcet's syndrome

Aphthous ulceration
Erythema nodosa
Orogenital ulceration
Pancytopenia and thrombosis
Thrombophilia

Churg-Strauss syndrome

Granulomatous lung disease
Mononeuritis multiplex
Pulmonary eosinophilia
Small vessel vasculitis (with granulomas)

Cirrhosis/chronic liver disease

Acanthocytosis
Ascites
Creatinine/urea ratio: raised
Eruptive xanthomata
Gynaecomastia
Hypoalbuminaemia
Hypoglycaemia
Hyponatraemia
Hypophosphataemia
IgA nephropathy
Lag storage curve
Low testosterone
Palmar erythema: causes
Pleural effusion
Raised AFP

Coeliac disease

Aphthous ulceration
Hyposplenism
IgA nephropathy
Protein losing enteropathy/malabsorption
Sideroblastic anaemia

Cushing's syndrome

Androgenisation
Hypertension in a young person
Hypokalaemic alkalosis
Myopathy
Osteoporosis

Diabetes mellitus

Abdominal pain and neuropathy
Abdominal pain (non-surgical)
Acidosis with raised anion gap
Autonomic neuropathy
Bilateral parotid swelling
Carpal tunnel syndrome
Chondrocalcinosis
Demyelinating changes on electromyogram
Hypermagnesaemia
Lag storage curve
Mononeuritis multiplex
Proliferative retinopathy
Renal failure with normal sized kidneys
Renal papillary necrosis
Secondary hyperlipidaemia
Third nerve palsy
Vibration loss
Vitiligo: associations
Xanthomata

Friedreich's ataxia

Absent reflexes with up-going plantars
Cardiomyopathy
Delayed visual evoked potential
Pes cavus
Retinitis pigmentosa
Spastic paraparesis
Vibration loss

Guillain Barré syndrome

Abdominal pain and neuropathy
Autonomic neuropathy
Bilateral facial nerve palsy
Bulbar palsy
Cerebrospinal fluid: raised protein with normal cells
Demyelinating changes on electromyogram
Motor neuropathy
Syndrome of inappropriate ADH

Haemochromatosis

Cardiomyopathy
Chondrocalcinosis
Chronic liver disease
Hypoadrenalism
Isolated hepatomegaly
Raised ferritin
Skin pigmentation

Histiocytosis X

Cranial diabetes insipidus
Fibrosis with normal lung volume
Granulomatous lung disease
Honeycomb lung
Primary sclerosing cholangitis

Hyperparathyroidism

Hypercalcaemia
Hypertension
Hypophosphataemia
Multiple endocrine neoplasia type 1
Multiple endocrine neoplasia type 2
Raised urate
Renal calcification

Hypoadrenalism

Hypercalcaemia
Hyperkalaemia
Hypermagnesaemia
Hypoglycaemia
Hyponatraemia
Raised urea: creatinine ratio
Vitiligo: associations

Hypoparathyroidism

Benign intracranial hypertension
Hyperphosphataemia
Hypocalcaemia
Papilloedema
Vitiligo: associations

Hypothyroidism

Acanthocytosis
Carpal tunnel syndrome
Galactorrhoea
Hypermagnesaemia
Hyponatraemia
Hypophosphataemia
Macrocytosis
Pleural effusion
Raised creatine kinase
Raised urate
Secondary hyperlipidaemia
Xanthomata

Inflammatory bowel disease

Aphthous ulceration
Clubbing
Erythema nodosum
Hepatic granulomas
Orogenital ulceration
Protein-losing enteropathy
Pyoderma gangrenosum
Ulcerative colitis: association
Uveitis

Iron deficiency

Anisocytosis
Dimorphic blood film (partially treated)
Howell-Jolly bodies
Microcytosis
Poikilocytosis
Target cells

Lead poisoning

Abdominal pain
Angioid streaks
Basophilic stippling
Cerebrospinal fluid: raised protein and normal cells
Demyelinating electromyogram
Macrocytosis
Motor neuropathy
Papilloedema
Sideroblastic anaemia

Lymphoma

Bilateral hilar lymphadenopathy
Bilateral parotid swelling
Cervical lymphadenopathy
Eosinophilia
Erythroderma: causes
Haemolytic anaemia: Coombe's positive
HIV and malaise/fever: nil focal
HIV and pancytopenia
Lymphocytes in cerebrospinal fluid
Mediastinal tumour: anterior
Paraproteinaemia
Protein-losing enteropathy
Pyoderma gangrenosum
Retro-peritoneal fibrosis
Superior vena cava obstruction

Motor neurone disease (anterior horn cell dise

Absent reflexes with up-going plantars
Axonal changes on electromyogram
Bilateral facial nerve palsies
Bulbar palsy
Pseudobulbar palsy
Small muscle wasting of hands
Spastic paraparesis

Muscular dystrophy

Creatine kinase: raised
Positive R wave in V1
Short PR interval

Myelodysplasia

Bone marrow failure
Macrocytosis
Pancytopenia and raised mean corpuscular volume
Sideroblastic anaemia

Myeloma

AL amyloid
Elevated erythrocyte sedimentation rate
Hypercalcaemia
Hyperuricaemia
Leukoerythroblastic anaemia
Pyoderma gangrenosum
Renal failure with normal renal size
Renal papillary necrosis

Myotonic dystrophy

Bilateral ptosis
Cardiomyopathy
Congenital cataracts
Left axis deviation
Polycystic kidney disease: associations

Osteogenesis imperfecta

Blue sclerae
Osteoporosis
Scoliosis
Short stature

Paget's disease

Angioid streaks
Bowing of the tibia
Frontal bossing
Osteopetrosis
Osteoporosis
Wide pulse pressure

Paroxysmal nocturnal haemoglobinuria

Abdominal pain: non-surgical
Haemolytic anaemia: Coombe's negative
Pancytopenia
Pancytopenia and raised mean corpuscular volume
Pancytopenia and thrombosis
Thrombophilia

Polio

Axonal changes on electromyogram
Bulbar palsy
Motor neuropathy
Pes cavus

Polyarteritis nodosa

Pulmono-renal syndromes
Roth's spots
Scleromalacia perforans

Porphyria

Abdominal pain and neuropathy
Abdominal pain (non-surgical)
Axonal changes on electromyogram
Motor neuropathy
Syndrome of inappropriate ADH

Pregnancy

Avascular necrosis
Carpal tunnel syndrome
Creatinine/urea ratio: raised
Galactorrhoea
Gingival hypertrophy
Hypercortisolaemia
Macrocytosis
Palmar erythema
Secondary hyperlipidaemia

Primary biliary cirrhosis

Chronic liver disease
Hepatic granulomas
Hypertrophic pulmonary osteoarthropathy
Isolated hepatomegaly
Secondary hyperlipidaemia
Ulcerative colitis: associations

Psoriasis

Erythroderma
Folate deficiency
High output heart failure
Hyperuricaemia
Koebnerisation
Onycholysis

Refsum's disease

Congenital cataracts
Nerve thickening
Retinitis pigmentosa

Renal tubular acidosis

Acidosis with normal anion gap
Osteomalacia
Renal calcification
Vitiligo: associations

Rhabdomyolysis

Creatine kinase: raised
Hypermagnesaemia
Hyperphosphataemia
Hypocalcaemia
Urea/creatinine ratio: raised

Rheumatoid arthritis

Aortic regurgitation: associations
Carpal tunnel syndrome
Mononeuritis multiplex
Osteoporosis
Psoriatic arthropathy
Pulmonary fibrosis
Pyoderma gangrenosum
Rheumatoid arthritis and renal failure
Scleromalacia perforans
Sideroblastic anaemia

Sarcoidosis

Autonomic neuropathy
Bilateral facial nerve palsy
Bilateral parotid swelling
Cardiomyopathy
Choroidoretinitis
Cranial diabetes insipidus
Dactylitis
Erythema nodosum
Hepatic granulomas
Hypercalcaemia
Interstitial nephritis
Leukoerythroblastic anaemia
Lymphocytes in cerebrospinal fluid
Mononeuritis multiplex
Nerve thickening
Renal calcification
Renal failure with normal sized kidneys
Syndrome of inappropriate ADH
Upper zone lung fibrosis
Uveitis

Sickle cell anaemia

Abdominal pain: non-surgical
Angioid streaks
Avascular necrosis
Dactylitis
Hyposplenism
Nephrotic syndrome
Proliferative retinopathy
Sickle cell and lung problems
Target cells

Sideroblastic anaemia

Basophilic stippling
Dimorphic blood film
Pappenheimer bodies
Raised ferritin

Silicosis

Bilateral hilar lymphadenopathy
Calcification of lung fields
Miliary shadowing on CXR
Pulmonary fibrosis

Syphilis

Absent reflexes with up-going plantars
Bilateral parotid swelling
Bowing of the tibia
Leukoplakia
Lymphocytes in cerebrospinal fluid
Orogenital ulceration
Saddle nose
Small muscle wasting of hands
Spastic paraparesis
Tunnel vision
VDRL: positive
Vibration loss

Syringomyelia

Pes cavus
Small muscle wasting of hands
Spastic paraparesis
Syringobulbia

Systemic lupus erythematosus

Anticardiolipin antibodies
Chorea: causes
Complement deposition and skin
Drug-induced lupus
Erythema multiforme
Haemolytic anaemia: Coombe's positive
Jaccoud's arthropathy
Livedo reticularis
Mononeuritis multiplex
Pancytopenia
Pancytopenia and raised mean corpuscular volume
Proliferative retinopathy: causes
Pulmonary fibrosis
Renal failure and low complement
Roth's spots
Scarring alopecia
Thrombophilia

Thalassaemia

Anisocytosis
Basophilic stippling
Frontal bossing
Microcytosis
Raised ferritin
Target cell
Tear drop cell

Thyrotoxicosis

Hypercalcaemia
Hypomagnesaemia
Lag storage curve
Osteoporosis
Pruritis
Pulse pressure: wide

Tuberculosis

Bilateral hilar lymphadenopathy
Bilateral parotid swelling
Calcification of lung fields
Cavitating lung lesion
Cervical lymphadenopathy
Erythema nodosum
Erythrocyte sedimentation rate: raised
Hepatic granulomas
HIV and malaise/fever (nil focal)
Hypoadrenalism
Intracerebral calcification
Leukaemoid reaction
Leukoerythroblastic anaemia
Lung abscess
Miliary shadowing on CXR
Protein losing enteropathy/malabsorption
Renal calcification
Renal papillary necrosis
Splenic calcification
Upper zone fibrosis
Uveitis

Tuberous sclerosis

Café au lait patches: associations
Fibrosis with normal lung volume
Honeycomb lung

Turner's syndrome

Atrio-septal defect
Coarctation of the aorta
Osteoporosis
Short stature
Ventriculo-septal defect

Waldenström's macroglobulinaemia

Erythrocyte sedimentation rate: raised
Paraproteinaemia: causes
Thrombophilia

Wegener's granulomatosis

Cavitating lung lesion
Pulmono-renal syndromes
Pyoderma gangrenosum
Saddle nose
Scleromalacia perforans

Wilson's disease

Chondrocalcinosis
Chorea
Chronic liver disease

Abbreviations

ACTH	adrenocorticotrophic hormone
ADH	antidiuretic hormone
AFP	alpha-fetoprotein
ATP	adenosine triphosphate
CXR	chest x-ray
DDAVP	desmopressin
DIDMOAD	diabetes insipidus, diabetes mellitus, optic atrophy and deafness
EEG	electro-encephalogram
ESR	erythrocyte sedimentation rate
FSH	follicle-stimulating hormone
G6PD	glucose-6-phosphate deficiency
GnRH	gonadotrophin releasing hormone
Hb	haemoglobin
HIV	human immunodeficiency virus
HLA	human leukocyte antigen
KCO	transfer factor
LH	luteinising hormone
MELAS	mitochondrial myopathy, encephalopathy, lactic acidosis and stroke-like syndrome
MPTP	1-methyl-4-phenyl-1,2,5,6-tetrahydropyridine
SXR	skull x-ray
TRH	thyrotropin releasing hormone
TSH	thyroid stimulating hormone
VDRL	venereal disease research laboratory